Crohn's Disease

The Ultimate Guide For The Treatment

& Relief From Crohn's Disease

By

Cailin Chase

Disclaimers

The information in this book is not intended as medical advice or a substitute for consultation with your healthcare provider. This information should be used in conjunction with the advice of your own healthcare practitioner. Always consult with your physician prior to changing and/or discontinuing medications or diet.

Any trademarks or product names used in this publication are the property of their owners, and are for identification only, and no claim implied by their use.

CONTENTS

INTRODUCTION

Crohn's disease is an inflammatory condition that can affect any section of the gastrointestinal tract. It is a condition that is becoming increasingly well understood by medical practitioners and the general public alike, but that said, this does not make receiving this diagnosis any easier. In particular, it is often confused for a disease known as ulcerative colitis. As such, this book aims to focus on helping you firstly gain a better understanding of the causes of Crohn's disease, the factors which influence its progression, and what you can do to regain your lost quality of life.

Not everyone gets diagnosed immediately, and this book will explain the whole process of getting a diagnosis and the different tests you may have to undertake in order to do so. An understanding of how Crohn's disease is diagnosed will also help reinforce your comprehension of how it develops in the first place. This knowledge will put power back in your hands to make informed decisions that will benefit you physically, mentally and even spiritually.

Crohn's disease is ultimately caused by a combination of many different factors and some of these relate to the immune system. Generally, immune-related diseases are difficult to treat in their entirety through conventional medical practice alone. To what extent this is down to lack of true understanding of the whole makeup of individual human beings as patients is debatable. In any case, you are probably all too aware that people with chronic diseases are often misunderstood. You will find that there is much to be gained in this respect from approaching an alternative practitioner.

Although great advances are happening all the time, resulting in new and improved treatment methods for all sorts of diseases, sometimes the medical community is guilty of considering patients as purely physical organisms without thinking of the person as a whole. This book aims to correct that approach by providing holistic advice from all sorts of reputable sources to supplement the support given by conventional treatment paradigms.

For thousands of years, we have known that all disease begins in the gut and what we choose to eat has a massive effect on our health as a whole. As such, a significant portion of this book will focus on dietary and nutritional changes you could make to improve your symptoms and reacquire your old way of life. To this end, a set of delicious recipes is included for you to get started on your journey towards better health.

CHAPTER 1 WHAT IS CROHN'S DISEASE?

Crohn's disease is an inflammatory bowel disease which can affect any part of the gastrointestinal tract. It is caused by a combination of factors including those environmental, bacterial and immunological in nature. The overall result is that the immune system attacks different portions of particular microorganisms, inadvertently affecting the body itself as well as the target.

Owing to the complexity of the combination of causative factors, it is not yet understood what the exact underlying issue within the immune system actually is. However, what is understood is that a significant proportion of the overall risk of acquiring Crohn's disease is ascribed to the involvement and effects of multiple genes on the immune system and gastrointestinal tract.

Each human being is unique, both from the biological perspective and from a more holistic standpoint. As such, when a disease is not completely understood it is all too likely that a conventional doctor may not get to the root of your problems. While a more holistic approach may not discover exactly why you are suffering the symptoms that you are, it will certainly aim to consider your existence as a whole rather than just making the simplistic assumption that you are just a collection of interacting organs.

The multitude of factors involved in the development of Crohn's disease means that symptoms may be gastrointestinal in nature or they may also include symptoms that you would not intuitively ascribe to ultimately having arisen as a result of a gut disorder. These symptoms will be considered individually in a later chapter.

For now we will focus on the different contributions towards the development of Crohn's disease that each causative aspect has to make. These factors may or may not exist in relation to every single person, and you may find that some combinations of causes apply to you whereas others do not. This merely goes to show that conditions such as Crohn's disease and thus the range of people suffering from it are really very individual and ought to be treated as such.

A significant proportion of blame can be placed upon your genetic inheritance for your having acquired Crohn's disease. More than 70 genes have been implicated in the disease and each of these plays a small but cumulatively important role in the development of your condition. This is particularly evident from the finding that if you have a sibling who suffers from Crohn's disease then you are 30 times more likely to develop it than a member of the general population.

At the present time, medical science has not progressed sufficiently for us to alter the effects of these faulty genes in a predictable and helpful manner. It is known that gene function can be altered, but as of yet little practical clinical benefit is possible.

Many of the inherited genetic mutations that can lead to Crohn's disease have to do with the immune system. For example, one such gene is known as NOD2 and its normal function is to promote the killing of a particular class of bacteria known as mycobacteria. The mutated form of this gene means that certain cells in your immune system, known as macrophages, are less proficient at killing this kind of bacteria. The result is that your body has poorer control of this kind of infection and this loss of control results in the chronic inflammation that is typical of Crohn's disease.

As mentioned, there are many genes which influence Crohn's disease and their biological function is known but for our purposes it is not necessary or helpful to dwell on the specific genetic components that have resulted in your individual form of the disease. However, the effects of this on the immune system should be considered briefly so that you can understand better the rationale behind particular treatments, whether conventional or holistic in nature.

In Crohn's disease the innate immune system, that is the aspect of immunity that is generalised and everyone has, is impaired. This means that the adaptive aspect of the immune system, the part that fights specific infections rather than having a general role, has to overcompensate. It is this overcompensation that results in a sustained microbe-induced inflammatory response. Though this can happen anywhere from mouth to anus, it most commonly affects the colon (large intestine) as this is where the greatest quantity of bacteria is found.

There is a theory that the increasing prevalence of conditions like Crohn's disease has to do with our modern hygiene habits, which when compared to earlier periods in human history seem rather excessive. We as a species evolved to cope with parasitic infections being a common occurrence, and the lack of this due to diligent hygiene practices means that our immune systems do not get enough practice, so to speak. Ultimately our immune systems are weakened, leaving us susceptible to immune-related disorders. In fact, upon being subjected to the presence of harmless parasites, human volunteers demonstrated an overall positive immune response. This is not to say that parasitic infection should be actively promoted, however.

Crohn's disease is typified by a weakened lining of the gut, known as the mucosal layer, as well as the inability to properly clear bacteria and other microorganisms from the natural pits in the gut wall. It is now thought that Crohn's disease may a actually be a number of different but similar diseases, dependent upon the exact species of microorganisms that is deemed causative in each case.

As previously mentioned, mycobacterium species are commonly implicated, but also E. coli is thought to be involved in a significant number of Crohn's cases. This is particularly important as this type of bacterium prevents your white blood cells from destroying dangerous bacteria in their normal way. The result is that bacteria live on within your cells themselves, causing inflammation and increasing the imbalance or dysbiosis of naturally present bacterial populations in your gut. It is precisely for this reason that dirt is thought to have a significant influence on the progression of Crohn's disease. It is hoped that with the help of the dietary advice in this book you will be able to drive our condition into remission and maintain this indefinitely.

There seems to be a clear link between the development of Crohn's disease and our modern lifestyles in industrialized countries. It may be that this is down to improved detection mechanisms and better diagnosis by well-informed physicians, but there are certainly a number of dietary and lifestyle factors that have a role to play in the development of Crohn's disease. These will be discussed in later chapters specifically dedicated to tackling this vast topic.

SIGNS, SYMPTOMS AND COMPLICATIONS OF CROHN'S DISEASE

As Crohn's disease is an immune-related condition rather than simply being a disease of the gut, there are vast range of potential symptoms not all of which involve the gut. Of course there are some symptoms which affect the gut exclusively, but there are also symptoms affecting other parts of the body as well as the body as a whole. This chapter aims to explain the different kinds of symptoms you might expect to come across.

Those symptoms which involve the gut in particular are known as gastrointestinal symptoms, and in Crohn's disease this means the whole gut from mouth to anus. Typically, though, symptoms result from the effects of Crohn's on the small and large intestines.

One of the first symptoms you might have experienced is abdominal pain which is common to all sorts of diseases and isn't really helpful on its own when working out what's going wrong. This may be accompanied by flatulence and bloating as a result of the inflammation and dysbiosis of normal gut flora. You can aim to reduce this aspect of your condition with dietary and lifestyle alterations as well as any advice or treatments that your conventional doctor might dispense.

Abdominal pain in Crohn's disease is usually accompanied by diarrhoea which can sometimes be bloody in nature. There is a positive side to the type of diarrhea that you experience in that it gives a clue as to which part of your gut is being affected by your disease at that time. When the small intestine (ileum) is being affected, the diarrhea tends to be more watery and occurs in high volumes. On the contrary, effects on the large intestine (colon) result in smaller volumes of diarrhea but at a higher frequency.

Diarrhea of this frequency can be inconvenient and if caught at the wrong moment it may be embarrassing. There is little one can say to alleviate this feeling but there are certainly things you can do in terms of your lifestyle to minimize the chance of diarrhea at an inopportune moment. This will be discussed a little later on, but for now remember that you can bring things under control with the right advice.

While it is possible that you may find blood in your stool if you suffer from Crohn's disease it is not cause for particular alarm in and of itself. In fact, visible blood in feces in not all that common in Crohn's disease and is more often associated with ulcerative colitis, so you may actually be able to use this finding to your advantage when getting a definitive diagnosis.

One of the consequences of chronic inflammation is that your intestines can become narrowed at specific points, a condition known as intestinal stenosis. Gastrointestinal symptoms are often at their most severe in Crohn's disease when this happens. You will likely find that your abdominal pain will especially intense when this happens and you may find yourself suffering from nausea and vomiting at the same time. It is at this time that surgery might be suggested to remove the small section of your gut that is affected. Although surgery can be a frightening prospect, nowadays such operations are quite routine and you will not be putting yourself at a high level of risk of complications.

As Crohn's disease may affect any section of the gastrointestinal system, you may find that you are affected by ulcers in your mouth. These tend to heal poorly without the intervention of a physician, so it is advisable that you go to your doctor for treatment in addition to following the advice of holistic practitioners. This may affect your ability to swallow properly, so you should try to consume only foods which are easy to swallow such as thick soups.

One of the more prominent symptoms of Crohn's disease has to do with discomfort and itching around the anus. This may be suggestive of inflammation or other complications such as abscess development and you might feel reassured if you pay a visit to your doctor to ensure that nothing untoward is going on.

As a result of anal involvement in Crohn's disease you may find you become prone to incontinence. Needless to say, this is not something that is at all comfortable or easy to deal with and may take some getting used to. It would be wise to be prepared for the worst when travelling anywhere, and having done so you ought not to have to worry excessively. If you are well prepared with a small selection of toiletries and a change of clothing, you can make steps towards living as much a normal life as possible.

As with many chronic inflammatory conditions, Crohn's disease can have effects on the body as a whole. Generally speaking, the systemic effects of Crohn's disease are caused as a result of the changes within the gastrointestinal tract and the behavioral changes that occur because of these changes.

Typically, people who suffer from Crohn's disease find that their symptoms ease off when they consume smaller quantities of food and this may lead to an overall loss in appetite. While this is perfectly understandable, it is important that you eat properly as Crohn's disease can quickly cause significant weight loss and malnutrition.

Those people who suffer from a particularly severe form of Crohn's disease affecting the small intestine may find that they lose weight at greater rate than might otherwise be expected from their decreased intake of food. This is because the majority of carbohydrates and fats are absorbed in the small intestine and Crohn's disease means that this process is severely impaired, resulting in malnutrition even when a proper, balanced diet is followed.

Poor function of the small intestine also may lead to the development of gallstones as bile acids are not properly resorbed and exit the body with stool instead. This alters the overall composition of fluids within the gall bladder, resulting in an increased risk of developing gallstones. Fortunately, this can be easily picked up by your doctor and is a particularly simple diagnosis to obtain. Treatment may involve surgery, but it is surgery of an absolutely routine sort and is undertaken daily all over the world.

Unfortunately, children suffer the consequences of the malabsorption and malnutrition associated with Crohn's disease in the form of growth failure. The positive side of this manifestation of the condition is that this is the way in which many cases of Crohn's disease are detected by doctors. At least when the cause is identified, you can start to work towards a solution to the problem of living with a chronic disease.

Owing to the vast number of genes involved in Crohn's disease, it comes as no surprise that other organs and bodily tissues can be affected by this condition. It is important to be especially aware of some of these conditions as the consequences of not treating them can be severe.

In particular, the various tissues that comprise the eye can be affected. Most commonly, the interior of the eye becomes inflamed in a disease known as uveitis. The result of this is blurred vision and pain in the eyeball particularly in the presence of light. The white of the eye may also be affected in a condition known as episcleritis. Both of these infections can result in the loss of eyesight if they are left untreated so it is always advisable to go straight to your doctor in the event that you notice anything unusual to do with your eyes.

Being that Crohn's disease is an immune-related condition, it is not surprising that it is associated with certain rheumatological diseases. Most commonly, Crohn's disease has been linked with a group of diseases which go by the umbrella term seronegative spondyloarthropathy. The essence of this collection of diseases is the inflammation of joints and the parts of the muscles that insert into the bones.

The symptoms commonly include painful and stiff joints which have become swollen and warm to the touch. Prolonged arthritis results in a loss of joint function as a result of reduced mobility. This can be particularly debilitating and may affect your quality of life considerably. Especially when it happens to younger people, not everyone in the general public understands the limitations that are placed on one's body as a result of arthritis of any kind. Hopefully with the right medications and holistic therapies you'll be able to minimize the effects of this aspect of Crohn's disease if it so happens to affect you. There's almost always something you can do to help yourself regain lost quality of life.

Generally speaking, there are two patterns that this disease might take. Firstly, the load bearing joints such as the knees, hips, wrists, shoulders and elbows may be affected. In the second variation of the two, the small joints of the hands and feet are affected in a symmetrical fashion. To satisfy diagnostic criteria, five or more of these small joints must be affected.

In some cases the spine may be affected and this aspect of the condition also comes in two flavors, so to speak. If the whole spine is affected by arthritis then this may lead to a condition known as ankylosing spondylitis, which is primarily characterized by an increasing rigidity of the spine. Alternatively, the arthritis may only affect one of the joints between the bottom of the spine and the hip (the sacroiliac joint).

The inflammation associated with Crohn's disease can also affect the skin and most commonly causes nodules to appear on the shins due to inflammation beneath the skin in this region. These nodules are raised, tender and red. Some nodules become ulcerated in nature and require delicate care to prevent further infection.

The generally pro-inflammatory state that your body is in as a result of the effects of Crohn's disease means that you are more likely to develop blood clots. It is important to be aware of this potential complication as blood clots can occur in the legs and in the lungs. In such an instance you may notice that one of your legs has become painful and swollen or that you are finding it increasingly difficult to breathe. In the event of such an occurrence you should immediately attend your nearest hospital to be examined and treated if necessary.

As a result of Crohn's disease you may be at increased risk of thinning of the bones, known as osteoporosis. This means that you may be more likely to fracture bones if you fall over or have some kind of physical accident. This risk is made worse by steroids prescribed to suppress your immune system to treat your condition, so you should be especially careful when out and about.

Owing to the nature of chronic disease as well as certain details specific to Crohn's such as intestinal blood loss and poor absorption of nutrients, you may find that you become anemic. Most commonly, this is due to a lack of iron in the diet or a loss of it due to minor but frequent bleeding from the gut. Vitamin B12 deficiency as a result of poor absorption of nutrients in the small intestine may also lead to anemia of a different sort.

While this vast list of symptoms seems daunting at best, the majority of people will not experience anywhere near all of these during their lifetime. The idea of this chapter is to just give you an idea of what could potentially happen so that you are at least aware of potential complications. We this knowledge in hand, you'll know what to do straight away if you experience any of these signs or symptoms. You can also take steps to alter your diet and lifestyle to minimize the chances of development of some of these complications. You may be further assisted by a holistic approach, examples of which will be shown in a later chapter.

CHAPTER 2 GETTING A DIAGNOSIS OF CROHN'S DISEASE

Getting a definitive diagnosis of Crohn's disease can be challenging to say the least and sometimes your doctor may not be absolutely 100% certain that this is in fact your diagnosis. As a result, going through the process of diagnosis and subsequent treatment can be a complicated and stressful process. It is hoped that armed with the knowledge in this book that you can take things into your own hands where it is appropriate to do so. Further knowledge on any topic can only be empowering and it is with this in mind that we proceed to a solution to your specific ailments.

Crohn's disease is often mixed up with ulcerative colitis before specific diagnostic tests are undertaken. This is simply because many of the features of each of these two diseases are very similar. However, there are certainly enough differences in most cases for your doctor to be able to work out what's going on.

The first thing a conventional doctor is likely to do when a diagnosis is not immediately apparent from physical examination and the symptoms you complain of experiencing is to order some blood tests. Unfortunately, when it comes to Crohn's disease most blood test results can only be used to diagnose a chronic inflammatory disorder involving blood loss or malabsorption. Nevertheless, certain blood tests are useful in making a diagnosis and assessing the effects of your condition. For example, iron deficiency anemia is common in all patients with Crohn's disease due to small levels of blood loss in the gut. As such your doctor will be looking for this and depending on its severity may recommend that you take iron supplements to increase your iron levels.

Another type of anemia can occur as a result of the malabsorption of vitamin B12 by the small intestine. This can be detected using a simple blood test and if present can be treated with supplements or some dietary alterations which we will discuss later on.

In order to check the overall inflammatory status of your body, you may have two blood tests done for acute and chronic inflammation. These tests are C-reactive protein (CRP) and erythrocyte sedimentation rate (ESR) respectively. If reported as high, this will help your doctor in diagnosing any inflammatory condition such as Crohn's disease.

As Crohn's disease is commonly mistaken for ulcerative colitis and vice versa, your doctor will often request a blood sample in order to test for anti-saccharomyces cerevisiae antibodies (ASCA) and anti-neutrophil cytoplasmic antibodies (ANCA). A test positive for ASCA and negative for ANCA is suggestive of Crohn's disease, whereas the opposite scenario is suggestive of ulcerative colitis. You do not need to remember these acronyms unless you really want to, but you should just be safe in the knowledge that there is a way to narrow down your diagnosis to the correct one even when several similar conditions are suspected. With this knowledge in hand, you can take steps towards treating your specific condition for your body.

One of the best ways to check for Crohn's disease remains the colonoscopy. This is a procedure involved a small length of tubing with a camera on the end. It is inserted in your back passage and allows your doctor to visualize the inflammation going on. Depending on the sort of inflammation present, your doctor may be able to make a diagnosis based on the findings of a colonoscopy alone. At present, about 70% of cases of Crohn's disease are definitively diagnosed in this manner.

It can be a difficult process to get a diagnosis and even then your lifestyle may be significantly impaired at least initially. Once you begin to come to terms with the kinds of lifestyle and dietary changes that need to be made, you can begin to work towards living a full life again. While you may find many activities inconvenient when you are having a flare up of your symptoms, most of the time you can enjoy a quality of life surprisingly close to what you would enjoy without the presence of Crohn's disease.

CONVENTIONAL TREATMENT

It is typically considered that there is no definitive cure for Crohn's disease owing to the significant genetic component. That said, it is admitted that you can push your condition into a state of remission. Having done so, many people find that they are able to maintain this state of remission for a significantly long period of time, sometimes even for years on end.

In order to do this, you may require the help of certain medications prescribed by your doctor. You can supplement any such treatment regime with lifestyle and dietary changes aimed at reducing inflammation and infection, thus reducing the symptoms of the disease and allowing you to live a more normal life.

There are several approaches taken by modern medicine in the treatment of Crohn's disease and these generally focus on the treatment of infections when they occur and the reduction of inflammation. Newer drugs have been developed to target the immune system itself, modulating its function to limit the progression of the disease process before chronic inflammation is allowed to take hold.

You'll often that you are being prescribed all sorts of antibiotics to combat the infections which lead to an exacerbation of your symptoms. While this is often necessary, it can have the unfortunate side effect of altering your gut bacteria such that you are even less able than usually to absorb the proper nutrients to keep your body fit and healthy. You can combat this detrimental effect by ensuring that you include probiotic and prebiotic foods in your diet wherever possible, providing that you do not experience discomfort upon consumption of certain products.

Your doctor will often prescribe anti-inflammatory drugs in order to reduce the effects of any flare ups in your condition. This may involve the use of steroids which should be taken with great caution. While they undoubtedly have a beneficial effect in that they suppress the immune system sufficiently to limit your symptoms, they have a global effect on the body resulting in a number of deleterious side effects. In particular, steroids such as prednisone can exacerbate the thinning of bones which you may already be experiencing as a result of Crohn's disease itself. As such, your doctor will likely only prescribe steroids for short periods at a time whenever possible.

An increasingly popular way to treat Crohn's disease is by modulation of the immune system. Rather than suppressing its functions in a general manner, this approach aims to limit the effects of certain aspects so as not to completely destroy the immune system's ability to fight disease. These use of these sorts of drugs can be discussed in depth with your doctor. Their potential side effects are not to be taken lightly, but they may well help you to treat your condition and get your life back on track. Drugs used in this way include methotrexate, azathioprine, infliximab, adalimumab and several others.

Owing to the gradual blood loss mentioned earlier, your doctor may wish to prescribe an iron supplement of some kind. If your deficiency is not too severe then they may suggest instead that you consume a greater quantity of iron-rich foods. This approach is advisable whenever possible as it is not wise to take too many medications when not absolutely required. The dietary section of this book will give examples of natural sources of iron.

In a minority of cases, surgical intervention may be warranted. It is important to note that this is not a curative treatment method, but can be used to relieve the effects of certain complications such as blockage of the intestines or development of abscesses.

As with any modern surgical procedure there is always a small risk involved but generally speaking complications are uncommon. Successive surgeries on the small intestine may result in what is known as short gut syndrome. This is where your small intestine is too short to be able to properly digest food and absorb nutrients. This will require nutrients supplementation under the guidance of your doctor.

HOLISTIC TREATMENT METHODS

There are a number of holistic treatment methods which have been used with great success in treating Crohn's disease. The best thing to do is to alter your diet and lifestyle, but there are also a number of other things that you can do to supplement this approach.

If you choose to pursue any form of alternative therapy it is always wise to inform your doctor of this before doing so. This way, your doctor can be made aware of any changes that might need to be made to your treatment regime. Often, conventional medicine is unable to fully treat a disease as it focuses primarily on physical symptoms. An holistic approach aims to consider you as a complete being with physical, psychological and spiritual aspects.

HERBAL MEDICINE

Before modern society developed, we humans had extensive knowledge of the many natural medicinal herbs and plants that are at our disposal. Nowadays we tend to use pharmaceutical medication to treat all of our diseases, but actually the majority of these medicines were first derived from plant sources that our ancestors would have made use of. This is most notably the case with painkillers such as aspirin and heart medications such as digitalis.

Given that plants contain similar forms of compounds as the drugs used by the modern pharmaceutical industry, it makes sense that certain plants can be used to great effect in the treatment of particular diseases. This is particularly true of Crohn's disease.

One of the most popular herbal remedies to use in the treatment of Crohn's disease and other inflammatory bowel conditions is aloe vera juice, which is known to have anti-inflammatory properties. Aloe vera has been used for many years to soothe all sorts of inflammatory ailments including burns, and you may well find that it has a calming effect on the bowels. It can be easily purchased in all health food stores.

The inner portion of slippery elm bark has been used by Native Americans for thousands of years in the form of a poultice with the aim of soothing injuries. It can be safely ingested, where it has a similarly soothing effect on inflamed bowels. Commonly it is made into a sort of gruel or porridge and flavored with cinnamon to gain an even greater anti-inflammatory effect.

Chamomile is known for its calming effects o the body even by the average member of the general public. It is commonly sold in the form of tea and is a delicious and easy way in which you can calm your whole body down, reducing stress and promoting the health of your gut and immune system. Speaking of teas and tisanes, green tea is an excellent beverage to consume for its health benefits and may help you to bring your disease under control.

Peppermint leaves are a great way to reduce cramping in the bowels, ultimately relieving you of a majorly disruptive symptom. With reduced abdominal discomfort, you'll find that you're able to enjoy more of the things in life that you used to. To double the benefit, you'll often find that green tea and peppermint are sold together as a blended tea.

A study undertaken in Germany has shown that consumption of a plant known as Boswellia has effects similar to the pharmaceutical drug mesalazine. Speak to your doctor first about this, but you may find that you are able to use Boswellia instead of certain medications ordinarily prescribed. As always with any powerful medication, whether herbal or pharmaceutical, really do make sure that you discuss things with your physician first.

Another plant that has been found to have soothing effects on the bowels is the marshmallow plant. This is the plant from which traditional marshmallows would have been made, rather than the kind of marshmallows sold today.

Whichever of these powerful herbs you try, make sure that you discuss it with your doctor in advance and of course also consult a qualified practitioner of herbal medicine. More and more doctors are becoming aware of the benefits of herbal supplements and medications, so you may find it extremely beneficial to speak with them about this. In fact, they may even be able to suggest you further treatments not mentioned here.

ACUPUNCTURE AND TRADITIONAL CHINESE MEDICINE

One of the major ways in which traditional Chinese medicine is having a positive influence on the Western approach to healthcare and medicine is to be found in acupuncture. It has been shown to be effective in the treatment of mild to moderate Crohn's disease, and is a holistic approach which takes into account all aspects of your individual being. Acupuncture makes use of very fine, sterilized needles to release endorphins, natural pain relieving, feel good hormones and compounds, and to affect the body's energy through the skin.

According to the philosophy underlying traditional Chinese medicine, the fundamental energy possessed by all living things is known as "Qi" and it is this vital force that is manipulated by means of acupuncture. It is considered that Qi runs through our bodies along channels known as meridians and that each organ is affected by the balance of this Qi. That is to say, an imbalance of any kind results in disease. The type of imbalance helps in the process of diagnosis and thus in the mode of treatment.

Qi is considered to have two opposing yet balancing aspects known as yin and yang. Generally speaking, rest corresponds to "yin" whereas activity corresponds to "yang". This concept is used in acupuncture alongside the concept of there being a five element system in nature.

The five elements of nature are represented by Wood and Fire as being more "yang", Water and Metal being more "yin", and Earth being a balance between the two. Each organ as a functional system is considered to be related to each one of these elements and an acupuncturist will assess overall health according to the effects of yin and yang on a person life force.

This is a gross simplification of the concept of traditional Chinese medicine but you can expect that diagnosis will made in part by means of feeling for a number of pulses on the wrist and tender points on the body, combined with a general enquiry about your health and state of mind. It is difficult to comprehend or even simply to accept this approach towards treatment for many of us in the Western Hemisphere, who are not accustomed to this kind of philosophy let alone this kind of medicine. Nevertheless, acupuncture has been shown to be of great benefit by robust studies conducted by reputable scientists.

There are four main theories as to why Crohn's disease occurs according to the ideas of traditional Chinese medicine. The first of which is the invasion of damp-heat in the large intestine. It is thought that this has to do with the overconsumption of fatty foods, a finding that is corroborated by Western medicine and anecdotal evidence reported by patients suffering from Crohn's disease. Reduction in consumption of these kinds of foods plus a course of acupuncture directed at stopping the disease process may be of great help to you.

The second theory speaks of a spleen deficiency, whereby the spleen is unable to function properly, leading to the disease states associated with Crohn's disease. As there is a significant immunological component the development of this condition, it does make sense that the spleen could be involved in some way. It is advised that you avoid cold or raw foods, particularly things like ice cream, in order to promote spleen health. This is also relevant in terms of reducing your dairy intake to prevent inflammation of the gastrointestinal tract.

Thirdly, spleen deficiency may be combined with kidney deficiency. As the kidneys are considered highly important in traditional Chinese medicine, being the root of all other organs and bodily processes, this particular issue is treated very seriously indeed. The approach to this kind ailment will generally be a prescription of specific herbs as well as a course of acupuncture. You should always consult your conventional doctor when taking additional medications of any kind so that they may be aware of any adverse interactions could occur as a result of mixing medications. Acupuncture is likely to be promoted by your conventional doctor as is something that is being increasingly accepted as a means to help control the stress associated with chronic disease processes.

The final of the four causes of Crohn's disease according to traditional Chinese medicine is the stagnation of Qi and the blood. This is frequently associated with the blood loss from the gastrointestinal tract attributed to the inflammatory effects of Crohn's disease. Acupuncture is used in an approach to treatment of this aspect of the condition by attempting to reduce the extent of blood loss as well as to reduce overall bodily stress. This may in part be effective due to the release of endorphins, the natural feel good compounds found within the body.

Regardless of how you personally feel about the approach taken by traditional Chinese medicine towards the diagnosis and treatment of disease, acupuncture as a treatment method has been shown to be useful in mild and moderate cases of Crohn's disease. You can always give it a go to see if it works for you.

AROMATHERAPY AND MASSAGE

Essential oils derived from all manner of fragrant plants have been used for thousands of years for their potential effects on illnesses. It has been increasingly shown by empirical scientific evidence that the properties of such oils known to our ancestors are genuine and can be used to effectively treat a range of diseases and symptoms.

Essential oils enter the body via the skin, and when you breathe in they have an effect on your sense of smell and are absorbed by your lungs and hence your bloodstream. Frequently this is accomplished by means of massaging the essential oils mixed with a carrier oil into the skin. Regardless of the medicinal effects of such oils, the act of having a massage in extremely relaxing in itself and may help to relieve some of the stress and anxiety that you have been feeling as a result of Crohn's disease.

The majority of essential oils used to treat digestive complaints such as Crohn's disease involve an attempt to reduce the spasms associated with it. As mentioned earlier in the chapter, chamomile and peppermint can be used effectively to this end. Other essential oils commonly used to reduce spasms and thus abdominal discomfort include clary sage, basil, yarrow and helichrysum.

Other essential oils such as lavender can be used for their purported effects on the nervous system which then have a knock-on effect on the digestive system by reducing spasms. Yet others are used for their overall anti-inflammatory effects such as turmeric which is well known in the Ayurveda medicine of India to promote the reduction in bowel inflammation as well to provide an anti-microbial effect. Of course, turmeric can be used to great effect in foods, particularly in those dishes originated from the Indian subcontinent.

CHAPTER 3 DIET AND LIFESTYLE ADVICE

Almost any disease process can be altered by the kinds of foods that you choose to consume, and this is particularly true of chronic inflammatory diseases like Crohn's disease. As the inflammation primarily affects your gastrointestinal tract it makes a lot of sense that what you consume has a significant influence on the health of the tissues with which it comes into direct contact.

There are a general set of rules that have been formulated based on a number of case studies, as well as some anecdotal evidence from patients who have suffered from Crohn's disease but were able to push it into remission and keep it there. It may appear unnecessarily restrictive to begin with, but you'll soon see that these particular rules have great merit and will almost certainly help you to bring your condition under control so that you can live a healthy and full life.

One of the first things to mention before we focus on the nutritional side of things is the issue of tobacco smoking. It has been conclusively proven that smoking worsens the symptoms of Crohn's disease and makes you more likely to suffer flare ups, so if you are a smoker then this is one thing that is under your control that you can give up in order to improve your health. Of course, this is easier said than done, but there are many support groups and sources of advice to help you quit smoking. For the sake of your quality of life, you can do anything you set out to do.

You should make sure that you consume plenty of water so that you can be sure that your bowels are kept clean and your body well hydrated. You would be well advised to choose water over other drinks such as coffee. The caffeine present in coffee and many other popular beverages has a stimulating effect on your gastrointestinal tract leading to worsening of symptoms such as cramps and diarrhea. Furthermore, you should avoid the use of certain artificial sweeteners, especially those based on sugar alcohols such as xylitol, as they also exacerbate diarrhea.

One of the major issues to do with formulating a diet plan suitable for Crohn's disease management is its fiber content. Some people find that a high fiber diet causes their symptoms to worsen. Often this feeling subsides and a high fiber diet becomes a key part of managing their disease. However, for others, fiber remains a problematic issue and should be avoided. You will know soon enough in which of these groups you reside. Sources of fiber include dried fruit, nuts, brown rice, beans and oats.

A high fat diet has been associated with exacerbation of the symptoms of Crohn's disease. In particular, fats of animal origin and polyunsaturated fatty acids have been implicated. As such it is advised that you obtain fats from sources such as oily fish and avocado. This will also help you to increase your intake of omega-6 fatty acids which have been shown to reduce your body's inflammatory state. You can do this also by taking fish oil capsules.

It has also been shown that the increased consumption of animal protein, as is typical of our industrialized societies, can lead to worsening of symptoms of inflammatory bowel diseases such as Crohn's disease. Despite this finding, you still need a protein source in your diet so the best options are to consume extra portions of fish which has no association with the progression of Crohn's disease. Furthermore, you can find a good protein source in vegetable products such as beans and pulses.

Some people have also reported that they suffer negative effects in the form of increased diarrhea and abdominal pain when they consume milk. This is thought to be due to the presence of the milk protein, casein. This is present in all dairy products and as such you may find it helpful to avoid dairy products entirely. This includes milk and cheese, but you may be able to tolerate butter as it is predominantly fat in its composition.

Similarly, gluten, a protein found in grains such as wheat, may exacerbate the symptoms of Crohn's disease. The general public is becoming increasingly aware of the effects of gluten on the body and as such you will be able to find all sorts of advice in books and other publications to help you choose foods or recipes that do not involve gluten-containing grains. In particular, this book contains a few example recipes that do not contain gluten.

Owing to the potential effects of Crohn's disease on the proper absorption of food, you may find that you have become anemic as a result of a deficiency of vitamin B12. This can be rectified with supplements or by consuming foods rich in this vitamin. Such foods fitting in with the rest of the dietary advice in this chapter include salmon and cod.

One of the best ways to influence your gut health through the modulation of gut flora is to consume prebiotic and probiotic foods. This will allow your gastrointestinal tract to function in a healthy manner conducive to a reduced level of inflammation, thus improving your quality of life.

Prebiotic foods are those which contain compounds such as fiber that cannot be broken down by the human body. Instead, they act as nutrient sources for beneficial species of bacteria in the gut. These bacteria promote the absorption of useful vitamins and minerals, something that of particular importance in Crohn's disease. Prebiotic foods include Jerusalem artichokes, garlic, leeks, onions and asparagus.

Probiotic foods are those which actually contain the beneficial bacteria which are needed to repopulate your gut in such a way as to promote the balance of gut flora and help with the absorption of nutrients. Usually a good source of probiotics would be fermented dairy products, but these ought to be avoided unless you find you can tolerate them without any worsening of your symptoms. Alternative, non-dairy sources of probiotics include sauerkraut and pickled cucumbers. A recipe for pickles is included in the cookbook section of this book.

Overall, you should try to make sure that your meals are frequent but small. This will allow you a chance to absorb as many nutrients as possible throughout the day without taxing your digestive system too much all in one go. If you can undertake some gentle exercise and improve your sleep pattern, then this will further enhance all of these dietary suggestions.

CHAPTER 4 COOKBOOK

This chapter is dedicated to giving you some examples of recipes following the dietary advice in the previous chapter. These recipes are designed to be relatively simple while maximizing the beneficial effects of each of the ingredients used. You will find recipes suitable for breakfast, lunch, dinner and snacks including smoothies.

EGG-WHITE OMELET WITH SMOKED SALMON, SPINACH AND CHIVES (serves 1)

- 1/2 tsp coconut oil

- 3 free range medium egg whites, gently beaten

- 1 1/2 Oz smoked salmon slices

- 1 handful baby spinach leaves

- 1/2 avocado, peeled and sliced

- 1 bunch of chives, chopped

- Pinch of ground black pepper

1) Melt the coconut oil in a pan over high heat.

2) Add the egg whites, stirring to scramble them for 30 seconds.

3) Allow the egg to settle in the pan, and add the smoked salmon slices.

4) Sprinkle the chives and spinach over the egg.

5) Season with black pepper and fold the omelet in the pan.

6) Serve with the avocado on the side.

ALOE VERA SMOOTHIE

- 1/4 cup fresh aloe vera, chopped

- 1/2 medium cucumber, chopped

- 1/2 medium banana, chopped

- 1/2 cup coconut milk (or other milk/milk replacement)

- 1/2 cup water

1) Blend all ingredients and serve immediately.

GRILLED PEPPERS (SERVES 4)

- 4 bell peppers, halved, seeded and stemmed

- 1/4 cup olives, halved and pitted

- 1/4 cup sun-dried tomatoes, rinsed and chopped

- 1 tbsp virgin olive oil

- 1 tbsp balsamic vinegar

- 1/8 tsp salt

1) Grill the peppers on a medium-high heat until soft and charred in spots. This will take about 5 minutes per side.

2) 2) Chop the peppers into cubes and mix them in a bowl with the olives, sun-dried tomatoes, oil, vinegar and salt.

3) Serve immediately.

CHICKEN AND LENTIL SOUP

- 1 tsp olive oil

- 1/2 medium onion, chopped

- 1 inch piece of root ginger

- 3 garlic cloves, chopped

- 2 green chilies (optional)

- 1/2 tsp ground turmeric

- 1 tsp salt

- 1/2 tsp ground cumin

- 5 oz split green lentils

- 2 pints organic chicken stock

- 3 1/2 oz chicken breast, skinned, poached and diced

- 1 tbsp lemon juice

- 2 tbsp fresh cilantro

1) Heat the olive oil in a saucepan.

2) Sauté the onion for 1 minute at a medium heat.

3) Add the ginger, garlic and chilies, and sauté.

4) Add the turmeric, salt, ground cumin, lentils and chicken stock to the saucepan. Cook at medium heat for 15 minutes. Pass through a sieve and return to the saucepan.

5) Add the diced chicken to the mixture, and bring it to the boil. Add water if necessary.

6) Simmer for 2-3 minutes and add the lemon juice.

7) Garnish with cilantro leaves.

POACHED SALMON FILLETS (SERVES 4)

- 1 pound salmon fillet, cut into 4 portions
- 2 tablespoons dry white wine
- 1/4 teaspoon salt
- 1 shallot, finely chopped
- Lemon wedges to garnish

1) Preheat oven to 220°C. Coat a suitable glass baking dish with cooking spray oil.

2) Place the salmon, skin-side down in the pan. Sprinkle over the wine.

3) Season with salt, then sprinkle over the shallots. Cover the fish with foil and bake until cooked in the center and starting to flake. This will take from 15 to 25 minutes.

4) When the salmon is ready, transfer it to dinner plates to serve. Spoon any liquid remaining in the pan over the salmon and serve with lemon wedges.

5) Serve alongside greens such as spinach.

SAUERKRAUT VEGETABLE MIX

- 1 quart sauerkraut, drained

- 1 onion, chopped

- 2 stalks celery, chopped

- 1 green bell pepper, chopped

- 1 large carrots, chopped

- 1 (4 oz) jar diced pimento peppers, drained

- 1 tsp mustard

- 1 cup sunflower oil

- 1/2 cup cider vinegar

1) In a large bowl, mix the sauerkraut, onion, celery, green bell pepper, carrot, pimento peppers and mustard. Set aside.

2) In a small saucepan, mix the oil and vinegar. Bring to the boil. Remove from the heat.

3) Pour the mixture over the vegetables and cover.

PICKLED GHERKINS

- 25 small cucumbers
- 1/2 lb. salt
- 2 quarts water
- 0.6 quarts white vinegar
- 1 tbsp pickling spice

1) Add the salt to the water to make brine.

2) Cover the cucumbers with the brine in a large pan.

3) Heat the liquid to near boiling point, but do not actually boil. Simmer for 10 minutes.

4) Drain the cucumbers and allow them to cool.

5) Place the vinegar and pickling spice in a saucepan and bring to the boil for 1 minute.

6) Pack the cucumbers into a warm Kilner jar, and cover with the vinegar.

SALTED ALMONDS (SERVES 2-4)

- 1 cup whole almonds

- 1 tbsp egg white, lightly beaten

- 1/2 tsp coarse sea salt

1) Preheat the oven to 350°F.

2) Spread the almonds on a baking sheet and roast for 20 minutes, until golden.

3) Mix the egg white and salt in a bowl. Add the almonds and shake well.

4) Tip the almonds back onto the baking sheet. Return them to the oven for 5 minutes.

5) Set aside until cold, then store in an airtight container.

BANANA AND RASPBERRY SOYA MILKSHAKE (SERVES 1)

- 1 banana
- 1/2 cup unsweetened soya milk
- 3/4 cup ice cold water
- 1/4 cup raspberries
- 1 tbsp coconut oil

1) Blend all the ingredients together and serve.

BASILMATO SANDWICHES

Ingredients:

- 4 slices bread

- 8-9 tsp. mayonnaise

- 4 slices tomatoes (thickly sliced)

- 4 tsp. basil sliced

- 1/8 tsp. salt

- 1/8 tsp. pepper

Method:

1) spread 2 tsp. of mayonnaise on each slice of the bread.

2) Top it with tomatoes, basil, salt and pepper.

GRILLED TOMATO SALAD

INGREDIENTS:

- 4 medium peppers, bell, halved, seeded and stemmed
- 1/4 cup black olives, oil cured, pitted and halved
- 1/4 cup tomatoes, rinsed and chopped
- 1 tablespoon olive oil
- 1 tablespoon vinegar balsamic
- 1/8 teaspoon salt

Method:

Grill the pepper on medium high for five minutes per side until soft. When cool enough to handle, chop the peppers into cubes and toss with olives, tomatoes, oil, vinegar and salt in a large bowl.

DELECTABLE SALMON FILLETS

Ingredients:

- 1 pound fish, salmon fillet, cut into 4 portions

- 2 tablespoons wine, dry white

- 1/4 teaspoon salt

- black pepper to taste

- 2 tbsp. shallots, finely chopped (1 medium)

- lemon, wedges, for garnish

Method:

1. Preheat oven to 425°F. Coat an 8-inch glass baking dish with cooking spray.

2. Place salmon in the prepared pan. Sprinkle with wine.

3. Season with salt and pepper, then sprinkle with shallots. Cover with foil and bake until opaque in the center and starting to flake, 15 to 25 minutes, depending on thickness.

4. When the salmon is ready, transfer to dinner plates. Spoon any liquid remaining in the pan over the salmon for better taste and serve with lemon wedges.

OVEN FRIES

Ingredients:

- 1 large potato, peeled and cut into wedges

- 2 tsp. extra virgin olive oil

- 1/4 tsp. salt

- 1/4 tsp. thyme (optional)

Method:

Preheat oven to 450°F. Toss potato wedges with oil, salt, and thyme (if using). Spread the wedges out on a rimmed baking sheet. Bake until browned and tender, turning once, about 20 minutes total.

Lasagna Rolls

Ingredients:

- 12 pieces Lasagna pasta

- 1 tablespoon extra-virgin olive oil

- 3 cloves garlic, minced

- 14 ounces tofu, extra-firm, water-packed, drained, rinsed, crumbled, (1 package)

- 3 cups spinach, chopped

- 1/2 cup cheese, Parmesan, shredded

- 2 tablespoons olives, Klamath, pitted, finely chopped

- 1/4 teaspoon pepper, red, crushed

- 1/4 teaspoon salt

- 25 ounces marinara sauce, preferably lower-sodium, divided

- 1/2 cup cheese, mozzarella

Method:

1. Boil water in a large pot and cook noodles according to the given package directions. Drain, rinse, return to the pot and cover with cold water until ready to use.

2. Meanwhile, heat oil in a large nonstick skillet over medium heat. Add garlic and cook, stirring, until fragrant, about 20 seconds. Add tofu and spinach and cook, stirring often, until the spinach wilts and the mixture is heated through, 3 to 4 minutes.

3. Transfer to a bowl; stir in Parmesan, olives, crushed red pepper, salt and 2/3 cup marinara sauce.

4. Wipe out the pan and spread 1 cup of the remaining marinara sauce in the bottom. To make lasagna rolls, place a noodle on a work surface and spread 1/4 cup of the tofu filling along it. Roll up and place the roll, seam-side down, in the pan. Repeat with the remaining noodles and filling. (The tofu rolls will be tightly packed in the pan.) Spoon the remaining marinara sauce over the rolls.

5. Place the pan over high heat, cover and bring to a simmer. Reduce heat to medium; let simmer for 3 minutes. Sprinkle the rolls with mozzarella and cook, covered, until the cheese is melted and the rolls are heated through, 1 to 2 minutes. Serve hot.

CREAM MUSHROOM SOUP

Ingredients:

- 5 cups mushrooms, assorted wild, (can also use shiitake, oyster, or regular white
- Mushrooms IF wild mushrooms are not available)
- 1/4 cup sherry (dry)
- 1/2 cup onions, red, minced
- 1/4 cup broth, chicken, fat-free, salt-free
- 1 teaspoon chives, minced
- 4 cups milk, fat-free evaporated
- 1/3 cup flour, all-purpose, unbleached
- 1 dash pepper, black ground

METHOD:

1) On a high medium heat, combine the mushrooms, sherry, onions and broth and cook them for five minutes until the mushrooms turn brown or golden.

2) Add the chives in the above ingredients and cook for two minutes. Add 3 ½ cups of the milk too. Lower the heat and simmer for five minutes.

3) Now combine the remaining ½ cup of milk and flour in the smooth and keep stirring it until it turns smooth and thick.

4) Add pepper to it and serve in a bowl.

STRAWBERRY-BANANA SMOOTHIE

INGREDIENTS:

- 2 cups strawberries, fresh, stemmed and halved (about 10)

- 1 1/2 cups soy milk, vanilla, low-fat

- 1 1/2 tablespoons honey

- 1/2 teaspoon vanilla extract

- 1 medium banana, sliced

- 1 cup whipped dessert topping, fat-free, thawed (optional)

- 2 sprigs mint, fresh, (optional)

Method:

Combine the strawberries, soy milk, honey, vanilla extract and banana in a blender, and process until smooth. Top each serving with whipped cream and garnish with mint sprig if desired. Serve immediately.

Linguine with Clams

Ingredients:

- 8 ounces pasta, linguine, uncooked
- 2 tablespoons oil, olive
- 2 cloves garlic, minced
- 1/4 teaspoon pepper, red, crushed
- 30 ounces clams, baby, canned, non-drained, (3 10-oz cans, such as Chicken of the Sea)
- 1/3 cup wine, dry white
- 1/3 cup broth, chicken, fat-free, salt-free
- 3 tablespoons parsley, fresh, chopped

Method:

- Boil the Pasta according to the package directions, omitting salt and fat.
- While the Pasta boils, heat oil in a large nonstick skillet over medium-high heat.
- Add Garlic and crushed red pepper, and sauté it for a minute or two.
- Drain clams, reserving juice. Add reserved juice, wine, and broth to pan. Bring to a boil; reduce heat to medium-high, and cook 5

minutes. Stir in clams; cook 1 minute. Stir in parsley. Toss with hot pasta.

PEPPY VIRGIN MARY

Ingredients:

- 2 cups juice, tomato, or vegetable juice, chilled
- 2 tablespoons lime juice, can substitute lemon juice
- 1 teaspoon Worcestershire sauce
- 1/2 teaspoon horseradish, prepared
- drops of hot sauce
- ice cubes
- celery, short stalks with leaves (optional)

Method:

In a small pitcher, stir together tomato juice or vegetable juice, lime or lemon juice, Worcestershire sauce, horseradish, and hot pepper sauce. If desired, serve over ice cubes. If desired, garnish with celery.

COCONUT APPLE CAKE WITH BROWN SUGAR

INGREDIENTS:

- 3/4 cup sugar, granulated

- 1/2 cup yogurt, nonfat, vanilla

- 1/4 cup oil, cooking

- 1 egg

- 1 1/2 teaspoons cinnamon, ground, divided

- 1 teaspoon vanilla extract

- 1/2 teaspoon baking powder

- 1/4 teaspoon salt

- 1/4 teaspoon baking soda

- 1/4 teaspoon ginger, ground

- 1/4 teaspoon nutmeg, ground

- 1 1/4 cups flour, all-purpose

- 1 pounds apples, Granny Smith, cored and coarsely chopped (3 cups)

- 1 cup coconut, flaked

- 3 tablespoons butter

- 3 tablespoons sugar, brown (packed)

- 2 tablespoons milk, fat-free

Method:

1) Preheat oven at 325°F. Line two 8x4x2-inch loaf pans with foil; coat foil with nonstick cooking spray. Set aside.

2) In a large bowl, stir together granulated sugar, yogurt, oil, egg, the 1 teaspoon cinnamon, the vanilla, baking powder, salt, baking soda, ginger, and nutmeg. Stir in flour just until combined. Fold in apples (batter will be very thick and chunky).

3) Spoon batter into prepared pans; spread evenly. Bake about 45 minutes or until a toothpick inserted near centers comes out clean and tops are browned.

4) Meanwhile, in a small saucepan, combine coconut, butter, brown sugar, milk, and the 1/2 teaspoon cinnamon. Cook and stir over low heat until the butter is melted. Preheat broiler after removing cakes from oven. Gently spread coconut mixture evenly over tops of cakes. Broil 4 inches from heat for 2 to 3 minutes or until topping is bubbly and lightly browned.

5) Cool cakes in pans on wire racks for 45 minutes. Use foil to lift cakes from pans; remove foil. Serve warm.

Pork Diane Recipe

Ingredients:

- 1 tablespoon water

- 1 tablespoon Worcestershire sauce

- 1 teaspoon lemon juice

- 1 teaspoon mustard, Dijon-style

- 4 Pork, boneless top loin chops

- 1/2 teaspoon lemon-pepper seasoning

- 1 tablespoon butter

- 1 tablespoon chives

Method:

1)For sauce, in a small bowl stir together the water, Worcestershire sauce, lemon juice, and mustard; set aside.

2) Trim fat from chops. Sprinkle both sides of each chop with lemon-pepper seasoning. In a 10-inch skillet melt butter over medium heat. Add chops and cook for 8 to 12 minutes or until pork juices run clear (160°F), turning once halfway through cooking time. Remove from heat. Transfer chops to a serving platter; cover and keep warm.

3) Pour sauce into skillet; stir to scrape up any crusty browned bits from bottom of skillet. Pour sauce over chops. Sprinkle with chives.

Power Burger Recipe

Ingredients:

- 1/2 pounds beef, lean ground

- 2 tablespoon oat bran

- 1/4 cup(s) oats

- 2 tablespoon milk, fat-free

- 1 teaspoon onion flakes, dehydrated

- 1/2 teaspoon oil, canola, or corn

- 1 dashes pepper, black ground

Method:

Mix beef, oat bran, oats, milk, onions and pepper all together and form into 2 patties. Deep fry the patties in oil in skillet and cook burgers until done.

LEMON PEPPER CHICKEN

INGREDIENTS:

- 3/4 cup(s) marinade, lemon-herb peppercorn, salt-free
- 12 ounce(s) chicken breast halves, boneless, skinless
- 2 cup(s) grapes, red
- 1 medium lemon, 4 wedges

Method:

1)Marinate the chicken breasts and place it on the unheated rack of a broiler pan. Broil 4 to 5 inches from the heat from 16 to 20 minutes until it   is   no   longer   pink.
2) For gas grill, place chicken on grill rack over medium heat and let it get grilled for 16-20 minutes.

3) Serve with grapes and lemon garnish.

TUNA SALAD

Ingredients:

- 1 large lettuce, green leaf, or red leaf

- 1/4 cup(s) celery, chopped

- tablespoon carrot(s), shredded

- 1/3 cup(s) fish, tuna, packed in water, drained tablespoon mayonnaise, light

Method:

Place the dried lettuce leafs on a serving table. Now mix celery, carrots, tuna, and mayonnaise in a small bowl and top lettuce leaf with tuna mixture.

Deli Turkey Roll up With Crisp bread and Grapes

Ingredients:

- 2 whole lettuce leaves, such as Romaine
- 3/4 ounce(s) turkey breast, roasted, sliced
- 1 tablespoon mayonnaise, light, divided
- 2 whole crackers, rye crisp bread
- 6 piece(s) grapes, seedless

Method:

Cut turkey into small pieces. Top lettuce leaves with mayonnaise and turkey and roll the lettuce leaves end to end. Enjoy the turkey roll-ups with crackers and grapes on the side.

WASHINGTON STATE APPLE BUTTER

INGREDIENTS:

- 2 ½ pounds apples, golden delicious, cored and cut into eighths
- 2 tablespoons lemon juice
- ¾ teaspoon cinnamon, ground
- ⅛ Teaspoon cloves, ground
- 1 tablespoon brown sugar

Method:

Combine the apples, ¾ cup water, and the lemon juice in a large nonstick pot. Bring to a boil over medium-high heat. Cover and simmer for 30 minutes.   Drain.

2) Push the apples through a food mill or strainer to puree and remove skin. Return the applesauce to the pot of water; add the cinnamon, cloves, mace, and brown sugar. Simmer over low heat until the mixture thickens, about   45   to   60   minutes,   stirring   often.

3) Cover and refrigerate. Apple butter keeps in the refrigerator for 1 week. Freeze for longer storage.

MANGO-STRAWBERRY SMOOTHIE

Ingredients:

- 1 1/2 cups orange juice

- 1/2 package tofu, silken-style firm, light

- 1 mango, pitted, peeled, and cut up

- 1 cup unsweetened whole strawberries

- orange sections

- mango chunks

Method:

In a blender, combine orange juice, tofu, the cut-up mango, and the 1 cup strawberries (If strawberry seeds are difficult for you to digest, substitute another fruit, like banana or blueberries) Cover and blend until smooth. If desired, for garnish, thread additional mango chunks, strawberries, and orange sections on 3 small skewers. Add a skewer to each serving. Serve immediately.

MINI MUSHROOM AND SAUSAGE QUICHES

Ingredients:

- 8 ounces breakfast turkey sausage, crumbled into small pieces

- 1 teaspoon olive oil, extra-virgin

- 8 ounces mushrooms, sliced

- ¼ cup scallions (green onions), sliced

- ¼ cup Swiss cheese, shredded

- 1 teaspoon black pepper, freshly ground

- 5 large eggs

- 3 large egg whites

- 1 cup milk, low-fat (1%)

Method:

1) Position rack in center of oven; preheat to 325°F. Coat a nonstick muffin tin generously with cooking spray.

2) Heat a large nonstick skillet over medium-high heat. Add sausage and cook until golden brown, 6 to 8 minutes. Transfer to a bowl to cool. Add oil to the pan. Add mushrooms and cook, stirring often, until golden brown, 5 to 7 minutes. Transfer mushrooms to the bowl

with the sausage. Let cool for 5 minutes. Stir in scallions, cheese and pepper.

3) Whisk eggs, egg whites and milk in a medium bowl. Divide the egg mixture evenly among the prepared muffin cups. Sprinkle a heaping tablespoon of the sausage mixture into each cup.

4) Bake until the tops are just beginning to brown, 25 minutes. Let cool on a wire rack for 5 minutes. Place a rack on top of the pan, flip it over and turn the quiches out onto the rack. Turn upright and let cool completely.

CRISPY POTATOES WITH GREEN BEANS AND EGGS

Ingredients:

- 1 cup green beans, fresh or cooked, cut into 1-inch pieces

- 2 tablespoons extra virgin olive oil

- 5 cups potatoes, cooked and diced, or 2 pounds boiling potatoes, peeled and cut into

- 1/2-inch dice

- 2 cloves minced garlic

- 1/8 teaspoon crushed red pepper

- 1/2 teaspoon salt

- Ground black pepper, to taste

- 4 large eggs

- 1 pinch paprika, (optional)

Method:

1) If using fresh green beans, cook in a large saucepan of boiling water until crisp-tender, about 3 minutes. Drain and refresh under cold running water.

2) Heat oil in a large nonstick or cast-iron skillet over medium heat

until hot enough to dazzle a piece of potato. Spread potatoes in an even layer and cook, turning every few minutes with a wide spatula, until tender and browned, 15 to 20 minutes for raw potatoes, 10 to 12 minutes for cooked.

3) Stir in the green beans, garlic, crushed red pepper, salt, and pepper.
4) Crack each egg into a small bowl and slip them one at a time into the pan on top of the vegetables, spacing evenly. Cover and cook over medium heat until the whites are set and the yolks are cooked to your taste, 3 to 5 minutes. Sprinkle the eggs with paprika, if desired, and serve immediately.

EGG AND SALMON SANDWICH

INGREDIENTS:

- 1/2 teaspoon extra virgin olive oil
- 1 tablespoon finely chopped red onions
- 2 large egg whites, beaten
- 1 pinch salt
- 1/2 teaspoon capers, rinsed and chopped, (optional)
- 1 ounce smoked salmon
- 1 slice tomato
- 1 whole English muffin, 100% whole-wheat, split and toasted

Method:

1) Heat oil in a small nonstick skillet over medium heat. Add onion and cook, stirring, until it begins to soften, about 1 minute.

2) Add egg whites, salt and capers (if using) and cook, stirring constantly, until whites are set, about 30 seconds.

3) To make the sandwich, layer the egg whites, smoked salmon, and tomato on English muffin.

PUERTO RICAN FISH STEW

Ingredients:

- 2 tablespoons olive oil, extra-virgin
- 1 medium onion, chopped
- 4 cloves garlic, minced
- 1 pound white fish (such as orange roughly, cod, haddock, or tilapia), cut into 1 ½
- Inch pieces
- 14 ounces tomatoes, diced
- 1 medium pepper or Anaheim, chopped
- ¼ cup cilantro, fresh, packed, chopped
- 2 tablespoons green olives, pimento stuffed, sliced
- 1 tablespoon capers, rinsed
- 1 teaspoon oregano, dried
- ½ teaspoon salt
- ½ cup water, as needed
- 1 medium avocado, chopped (optional)
- Leave out the tomatoes and peppers if these foods cause problems for you.

Method:

1) Heat oil in a large high-sided skillet or Dutch oven over medium heat. Add onion and cook, stirring occasionally, until softened, about 2 minutes.

2) Add garlic and cook, stirring, for 1 minute.

3) Add fish, tomatoes and their juices, Chile pepper, cilantro, olives, capers, oregano and salt; stir to combine. Add up to ½ cup water if the mixture seems dry.

4) Cover and simmer for 20 minutes. Remove from the heat.

5) Serve warm or at room temperature, garnished with avocado (if using).

VERSATILE VEGETABLE SOUP

Ingredients:

- 3 leeks, thinly sliced (white parts only)
- 1 1/2 teaspoon minced garlic
- 1 teaspoon olive oil
- 8 cups water
- 14 1/2 ounces stewed tomatoes
- 4 stalks celery, sliced
- 3 medium carrots, thinly sliced
- 1 medium apple, cored and coarsely chopped
- 1 medium sweet potato, peeled and cut into 1/2-inch cubes
- 4 teaspoon vegetable bouillon
- 2 cups red cabbage, shredded
- 1 cup green beans
- 1/4 teaspoon salt
- 1/4 teaspoon black ground pepper
- 1/2 cup parsley
- 2 tablespoons lemon juice

Method:

In a 4-quart Dutch oven, cook leeks and garlic in hot oil about 3 minutes or until nearly tender. Carefully add the water, non-drained tomatoes, celery, carrots, apple, sweet potato, and bouillon granules or cubes. Bring to boiling; reduce heat. Cover and simmer for 15 minutes. Add cabbage, green beans, salt, and pepper. Return to boiling; reduce heat. Cover and simmer about 10 minutes more or until vegetables are tender. Stir in parsley and lemon juice.

ROASTED POTATOES AND BABY CARROTS

Ingredients:

- 1 tablespoon olive oil

- 1 bag baby carrots (1-pound)

- 1 pound red potatoes, small, quartered

- 1 teaspoon thyme, fresh, leaves only

Method:

1) Preheat the oven to 400 degrees F.

2) Brush a rimmed baking sheet lightly with oil.

3) Place carrots and potatoes, cut side down, on the baking sheet. Drizzle with oil and sprinkle with thyme, salt and pepper. Toss to lightly   coat.

4) Roast for 15 minutes, remove from the oven and stir to combine. Roast for 10-15 minutes or until vegetables turn tender and slightly charred.

Artichoke and Ripe-Olive Tuna Salad

INGREDIENTS

- 12 ounces light tuna fish, packed in water, drained and flaked
- 1 cup artichoke hearts
- 1/2 cup olives, pitted, chopped
- 1/3 cup reduced-fat mayonnaise
- 2 teaspoons lemon juice
- 1 1/2 teaspoons fresh oregano, chopped or 1/2 teaspoon dried

Method:

Put the ingredients; tuna, artichokes, olives, mayonnaise, lemon juice, and oregano in a medium bowl and mix it properly. Now serve with fresh salad leaves.

Juicy Hamburger Buddy

Ingredients:

- 3cloves garlic, crushed and peeled
- 2 medium carrots, cut into 2-inch pieces
- 10 ounces mushrooms, white, large, cut in half
- 1 large onion, cut into 2-inch pieces
- 1 pound beef, lean ground, 90% lean
- 2 teaspoons thyme, dried
- ¾ teaspoon salt
- ¼ teaspoon black ground pepper
- 2 cups water
- 14 ounces beef broth, low sodium, divided
- 8 ounces pasta, whole-wheat, elbow macaroni
- 2 tablespoons Worcestershire sauce
- 2 tablespoons flour, all-purpose
- ½ cup sour cream, reduced-fat
- 1 tablespoon parsley, chopped (or chives)

Method:

1) Fit a food processor with the steel blade attachment. With the motor running, drop garlic through the feed tube and process until minced, and then add carrots and mushrooms and process until finely chopped. Turn it off, add onion, and pulse until roughly chopped and forms a proper paste.

2) Cook beef in a large straight-sided skillet or Dutch oven over medium-high heat, breaking it up with a wooden spoon, until no longer pink for at least 3 to 5 minutes.

3) Stir in the chopped vegetables, thyme, salt and pepper and cook, stirring often, until the vegetables start to soften and the mushrooms release their juices, 5 to 7 minutes.
4) Stir in water, 1 ½ cups broth, noodles and Worcestershire sauce; bring to a boil. Cover; reduce heat to medium and cook, stirring occasionally, until the pasta is tender, 8 to 10 minutes.

5) Whisk flour with the remaining ¼ cup broth in a small bowl until smooth; stir into the hamburger mixture. Stir in the sour cream. Keep stirring the sauce for at least 3-5 minutes until it smoothens and form a paste. Serve sprinkled with parsley (or chives), if desired.

GRILLED EGGPLANT PARMESAN SANDWICH

Ingredients:

- 1 large eggplant, (1.25-1.5-pounds), cut into 12, 1/4-inch thick rounds
- Olive oil-flavored cooking spray, to coat eggplant
- 1/4 teaspoon salt
- 3 tablespoons cheese, finely shredded Parmesan
- 1/2 cup part-skim shredded mozzarella cheese
- 4 pieces focaccia or rustic Italian bread
- 2 teaspoons extra virgin olive oil
- 5 ounces baby spinach
- 1 cup crushed tomatoes, preferably fire-roasted
- 3 tablespoons fresh basil, chopped, divided

Method:

1. Preheat grill to medium-high.

2. Place eggplant rounds on a baking sheet and sprinkle with salt. Coat both sides lightly with cooking spray. Combine Parmesan and mozzarella in a small bowl. Brush both sides of Focaccia (or bread) with oil.

3. Place spinach in a large microwave-safe bowl. Cover with plastic wrap and punch several holes in the wrap. Microwave it for 2 to 3 minutes until wilted. Combine tomatoes and 2 tablespoons basil in a small microwave-safe bowl. Cover and microwave until bubbling, about 2 minutes.

4. Place all your ingredients on the baking sheet with the eggplant and take it to the grill. Grill the eggplant slices until brown and soft on both sides, 2 to 3 minutes per side. Grill the bread until toasted, about 1 minute per side. Return the eggplant and bread to the Baking sheet. Reduce grill heat to medium.

5. Place 1 eggplant round on top of each slice of bread. Layer 1 tablespoon tomatoes, 1 tablespoon wilted spinach, and 1 tablespoon cheese on each slice of eggplant.

PORK CHOPS WITH PEACH BARBECUE SAUCE

Ingredients:

- 1/4 cup kosher salt

- 1/4 cup brown sugar, (packed)

- 2 cups boiling water

- 3 cups ice cubes

- 4 pieces trimmed center-cut pork chops, bone-in, 1/2-3/4 inch thick, (1 3/4-2 pounds)

- 2 large peaches, ripe but firm, pitted and quartered, or 3 cups frozen sliced peaches

- 1/2 teaspoon salt, Kosher

- 1 medium tomato, quartered and seeded

- 2 tablespoons cider vinegar

- 1 tablespoon canola oil

- 1/2 cup onions, chopped, preferably Vidalia

- 2 teaspoons ginger, fresh, finely chopped

- 2 tablespoons honey

1/4 teaspoon pepper, black ground, plus more to taste

Method:

1) Place 1/4 cup salt and brown sugar in a medium heatproof bowl. Pour in boiling water and stir to dissolve. Add ice cubes and stir to cool. Add pork chops, cover and refrigerate for at least 30 minutes or up to 4 hours.

2) Puree peaches, tomato, and vinegar in a food processor until smooth.

3) About 30 minutes before you're ready to cook the pork chops, heat oil in a medium saucepan over medium-high heat. Add onion and cook, stirring occasionally, until golden brown, 5 to 7 minutes.

4) Add ginger and cook, stirring frequently, until fragrant, 1 to 2 minutes.

Add the peach puree, the remaining 1/2 teaspoon salt, honey, and pepper to taste. Bring to a boil over high heat, and then reduce the heat to a simmer. Cook until reduced by about half, 20 to 25minutes. Reserve 1/4 cup of the sauce for basting the chops; keep the remaining sauce warm in the saucepan until ready to serve.

5. Preheat grill to medium.

6. Remove the pork chops from the brine (discard brine), rinse well, and thoroughly dry with paper towels. Season the chops with 1/4 teaspoon pepper and brush both sides with some of the reserved sauce.

7. Grill the pork chops, turning once, until an instant-read thermometer inserted into the center registers 145°F, 2 to 4 minutes per side. Transfer

to a plate, tent with foil, and let rest for 5 minutes. Serve with the warm

peach barbecue sauce on the side

CHICKEN-TOFU STIR-FRY

Ingredients:

- 2 tablespoons olive oil
- 2 tablespoons orange juice
- 1 tablespoon reduced-sodium soy sauce
- 1 tablespoon Worcestershire sauce
- 1 tablespoon fresh ginger or 1 teaspoon ground ginger
- 1 teaspoon dry mustard
- 1 teaspoon turmeric
- 8 ounces chicken breast (cooked), cubed
- 8 ounces tub-style extra firm tofu, drained and cubed
- 2 medium carrots, bias-sliced or 2 stalks celery, thinly sliced
- 1 cup fresh mushrooms, sliced, and/or fresh or frozen, thawed pea pods
- 3 cups brown rice, cooked
- 3 scallions (green onions), cut into 1/2-inch-long pieces
- 1 medium red or green bell pepper, cut into thin bite-size strips
- 1Cups baby bock Choy, chopped, and/or fresh bean sprouts

Method:

1. In a large bowl, stir together 1 tablespoon of the oil, the orange juice, soy sauce, Worcestershire sauce, ginger, mustard, and turmeric. Add cooked chicken and tofu cubes; stir to coat. Cover and marinate in the refrigerator for 1 to 4 hours.

2. In a very large nonstick skillet, heat remaining 1 tablespoon oil over medium-high heat. Add carrot or celery; cook and stir for 2 minutes. Add mushrooms and/or pea pods; cook and stir for 2minutes. Add bock Choy and/or bean sprouts, green onions, and sweet pepper; cook and stir for 2 minutes. Add non drained chicken mixture; heat through. Serve with hot cooked rice.

Brown Rice and Tofu Maki

Ingredients:

- 4 1/4 cups water
- 2 1/4 cups short-grain brown rice
- 3 tablespoons miring (sweet rice wine)
- 3 tablespoons reduced-sodium soy sauce
- 3 1/2 teaspoons sugar, divided
- 1/3 cup rice vinegar
- 1/2 teaspoon salt
- 8 sheets toasted nori seaweed (wakame)
- 32 slices ready-to-eat, teriyaki flavored, or Thai tofu, baked, cut into matchstick strips
- 32 slices red bell peppers, (about 1 small pepper) cut into matchstick strips
- 32 slices cucumbers, peeled, seeded, (about 1/2 small cucumber) cut into matchstick strips
- 4tablespoons unsalted roasted peanuts, crushed

Method:

3) Bring water to a boil in a large saucepan over medium heat. Stir in rice, reduce heat to low, cover, and simmer at the lowest bubble until the rice is tender, about 50 minutes. Remove from the heat and let stand, covered, for 10 minutes.

4) Meanwhile, stir mirin, soy sauce, and 1 1/2 teaspoons sugar in a small skillet. Bring to a simmer and cook until slightly thickened, about 3 minutes.

5) Spread the warm rice evenly on a large rimmed baking sheet. Whisk vinegar, the remaining 2 teaspoons sugar, and salt in a small bowl; drizzle over the rice. Toss with 2 spatulas until cool enough to handle and slightly sticky.

6) Place a nori sheet on a bamboo sushi-rolling mat-shiny side down with a shorter end close to you. Wet your hands and pat about 3/4 cup of the seasoned rice into a thin layer on the sheet, leaving a1-inch border at the top of the sheet (the short side on the far side of the mat).

7) Drizzle 1 teaspoon of the mirin sauce about 1 inch from the bottom of the rice; place 4 strips each baked tofu, bell pepper, and cucumber over the sauce; then sprinkle with about 2 teaspoons chopped peanuts.

8) Using the bamboo mat to help you, roll the maki closed, getting the mat out from inside the maki as it rolls up. Gently press the closed mat over the roll to seal the roll. Trim any ragged edges and slice into 6 pieces with a wet sharp knife.

9) Repeat Step 4 with the remaining nori, rice, tofu, and vegetables. Serve the rolls with any remaining sauce.

BANANA RICE PUDDING

Ingredients:

- 1 cup brown basmati rice

- 2 cups water

- 1/2 teaspoon salt

- 4cups gluten-free vanilla ice milk

- 1 teaspoon gluten-free vanilla ice milk

- 1/3 cup light brown sugar

- 1/2 teaspoon ground cinnamon, plus more for garnish

- 1 tablespoon cornstarch

- 4 medium ripe bananas, divided

- 1 teaspoon vanilla extract

Method:

1. Combine rice, water, and salt in a medium saucepan and bring to a boil. Reduce heat to low, cover, and cook until the liquid is fully absorbed, 45 to 50 minutes.

2. Stir in 3 cups rice milk, brown sugar, and 1/2 teaspoon cinnamon and bring to a lively simmer. Cook for 10 minutes while stirring occasionally.

3. Stir cornstarch and the remaining 1 tablespoon rice milk in a small bowl until smooth; add to the pudding. Continue cooking, stirring often, until the mixture is the consistency of porridge, about 10 minutes. Remove from the heat.

4. Mash 2 bananas in a small bowl. Stir the mashed bananas and vanilla into the pudding.

5. Transfer to a large bowl, cover and refrigerate until cold, at least 2 hours.

6. Just before serving, slice the remaining 2 bananas. Top each serving with a few slices of banana and sprinkle with cinnamon, if desired.

MASHED POTATOES.....................

Ingredients:

- 2 Potatoes, boiled and peeled off

- Water

Method:

1) Boil the two potatoes in a saucepan in 4 glass of water until turn soft.

2) Peel the off and mash them properly until no bulk found.

3) Serve in a bowl.

WHOLE-GRAIN PANCAKES WITH APRICOT RICOTTA

Ingredients:

- 1 cup self-rising whole-grain flour

- 1 tablespoon sugar

- 1/4 cup skim milk powder

- 1 egg

- 1/2 cup skim (or low-fat) milk

- 1/4 teaspoon baking soda

- Canola margarine for cooking the pancakes

- 8 ounces ricotta cheese

- 1/2 tablespoon honey

- 1 cup canned apricots in their juice

Method:

1) Combine flour, sugar, and skim milk powder in bowl. Add egg, milk, and baking soda, and whisk until smooth.

2) Heat the frying pan to medium-high heat and melt a small amount of canola margarine in it to coat the pan. Pour in 1/4 of the batter to

make 2 small pancakes.

3) Cook until bubbles form, then flips to cook other side of the pancake. Repeat until you have 8 small pancakes.

APRICOT RICOTTA:

Puree ricotta with honey and canned apricots until smooth. Serve apricot ricotta over double-stacked pancakes. Eat immediately.

GLUTEN-FREE TOMATO BASIL PASTA

Ingredients:

- 1 cup canned chopped tomato (with juices)
- 2 tablespoons extra virgin olive oil
- 2 tablespoons large sliced garlic
- Pinch kosher salt
- Pinch crushed black pepper
- Large pinch basil (medium chop)
- 6 wt. ounces gluten-free capelin, spaghetti or linguine

Method:

1) Place tomatoes with their juice in a sauté pan.

2) In a separate sauté pan, the heat garlic and extra virgin olive oil over a low flame, stirring occasionally. Cook to soften garlic and release flavor into the oil. Do not brown the garlic or it will overcook. Let garlic and oil mixture cool.

3) Add the tomatoes with their juices mixture along with the salt and pepper to the garlic and oil. Stir until thoroughly mixed. Add the basil and stir again. Return flame to medium low.

4) Cook the pasta in boiling, salted, water until cooked. Drain well and add to the sauce.

5) Toss the pasta with the sauce and serve in a pasta bowl.

RAINBOW WRAP

Ingredients:

- 1 tablespoon hummus

- 1 whole-grain pita or wrap

- 1 leaf of lettuce, shredded

- 1 whole canned or cooked beet, chopped

- 1 small cooked sweet potato, cooled

- 1/2 medium tomato, seeded—also add several chopped up dried tomatoes if tolerated

- 1/4 cup basil leaves

- 1 ounce reduced-fat feta cheese (or 1 hard-boiled egg)

- 1 shallot, chopped (optional)

Method:

Spread hummus over pita or wrap and cover with lettuce. Place canned or cooked beet, booked sweet potato, tomato, basil leaves, and cheese along one half of the wrap and roll up. Have plastic cling wrap ready to wrap it. Slice in half and pack for work.

CHICKEN AND VEGETABLE PIZZA

Ingredients:

- 1 medium sweet potato, sliced and sprayed with olive oil

- 1 1/2 cups zucchini, sliced and sprayed with olive oil

- 1 1/2 cups red bell pepper, sliced into quarters and sprayed with olive oil

- 2 tablespoons olive oil

- 12 ounces skinless chicken breast fillet

- Lemon juice, to taste

- Pepper, to taste

- 2 thin, frozen medium-sized pizza crusts

- 1/2 cup tomato paste, canned or homemade (reduce 1 1/2 cups crushed canned tomato on stove)

- 2 cloves of garlic, crushed

- 2 ounces low-fat feta cheese, cut into 1/2-inch cubes

- 1 cup fresh basil

- 1 tablespoon pine nuts (optional)

- 2 sprigs fresh (or dried) rosemary (optional)

- 1/2 cup Parmesan cheese (optional)

Method:

1)   Preheat   the   oven   at   350   degree   Celsius.

2) Place sweet potato, zucchini, and red bell pepper on a tray. Place in a 350° oven for half an hour, turning once. While baking, use 1 tablespoon of olive oil in a pan to sauté chicken in lemon juice and pepper   until   nearly   cooked.

3) Remove from pan and cut chicken into bite-sized chunks. Grease top of pizza crust with oil and spread tomato paste over the crusts. Sprinkle with garlic and then layer baked vegetables and chicken pieces onto the pizza

4) Add small pieces of feta cheese and torn-up basil. Sprinkle with pine nuts, rosemary, and Parmesan cheese, as desired.

Bake at 400° F for 10 to 15 minutes.

Pesto Pasta Salad

INGREDIANTS

- 2 cups dry pasta spirals or suitable shapes (if using rice, use 1 cup dry rice)
- 24 small cherry tomatoes, cut in halves
- 20 black olives (pitted)
- 1 cup snow peas
- 8 ounces lean lunch-meat slices; or skinless cooked chicken, cubed; or tuna chunks
- 2 cups mixed green leaves
- 1 cup walnut pesto

METHOD

Cook pasta or rice at least an hour in advance, and cool in refrigerator. Make pesto just before assembling salad, and mix with pasta (or rice). Combine all ingredients in a large salad bowl just before serving.

GREEN VEGGIE CUTLETS

INGREDIANTS:

- 1 medium potato

- 1 medium sweet potato

- 2 medium carrots

- 2 medium zucchini

- 2 cups chopped broccoli

- 2 tablespoons chopped spring onions or chives

- 2 tablespoons chopped walnuts or whole pine nuts

- 2 eggs, beaten

- 2 tablespoons soy flour (or whole-grain wheat flour)

- Canola oil

Method:

1)Use a food processor or grater to shred potato, sweet potato, carrots, and zucchini. Press excess water out of the shredded vegetables and pour off liquid.

2) Mix shredded vegetables thoroughly and add finely chopped broccoli, chopped spring onions or chives, and walnuts or pine nuts. Add beaten eggs and flour, and mix thoroughly.

3) Put small amounts of the mixture slowly into heavy frying pan. Press mixture out into patties of pancake thickness. Cook on medium heat for 5 minutes on each side, until golden.

4) You can make 12 patties. Make a stack of 3 and serve beside the salmon.

Vanilla Chiffon Cake

INGREDIANTS:

- 1 1/4 cup rice flour (white or brown)
- 1 cup sugar
- 1 1/2 teaspoon double acting baking powder (gluten-free)
- 1/2 teaspoon salt
- 1 1/3 cup milk (cow, rice or soy)
- 1/3 cup shortening
- 1 egg
- 1 teaspoon vanilla
- 1 1/2 teaspoon egg substitute powder mixed with 2 tablespoons warm water
- 1 tablespoon lemon juice

Method:

1) Spray inside of a microwavable cake pan with non-stick cooking spray and dust with corn meal.

2) Mix all ingredients, except the egg substitute powder and lemon juice, in a large mixing bowl. Use mixer set on lowest speed and beat for one minute.

3) Mix the egg substitute powder with warm water and add it and lemon juice to cake batter. Set mixer on high and beat for three more minutes.

4) Pour cake batter into prepared pan and immediately microwave on high for 5 to 7 minutes. Position cake pan on outer edge of the microwave carousel, otherwise, the center will not thoroughly cook.

5) Allow cake to cool for 5-10 minutes before inverting onto a cooling rack.

Variations and Extras:

A one layer orange chiffon cake is achieved by adding 3 teaspoons of real orange juice and orange zest to the batter. To make a chocolate version of the cake add cocoa or melted chocolate to the batter.

Ideas for frosting: Sprinkle powdered sugar, layer with jam or jelly, or decorate with real fruit.

YUMMILICIOUS MEATBALLS

Ingredients:

- 8 ounces lean minced beef

- 8 ounces lean minced lamb

- 1 cup cooked rice (let cool before using)

- 1 tablespoon milk

- 1 beaten egg

- 1 teaspoon Italian herbs or tolerated Asian herbs

- 1/2 tablespoon favorite mild mustard

- Freshly ground black pepper, amount desired

- Canola oil

Method:

Mix all ingredients except canola oil in a bowl. Wet hands and make golf-ball-sized meatballs. Refrigerate until ready. Use canola oil to lightly coat the pan, and then fry meatballs gently. Avoid cooking for more than 2 to 3 minutes on any side, and turn balls over at least 3 times. Meatballs should be tender but cooked through. Place meatballs on toothpicks or thread along 4 skewers to serve.

Make this dipping sauce if tomatoes are tolerated:

1)15-ounce can crushed tomatoes

2) Fresh chopped basil, or dried basil, or 1 tablespoon sweet chili sauce if tolerated

3) Heat crushed tomatoes in saucepan. Reduce to desired consistency. Stir in basil or sweet chili sauce during the final minutes.

DATE SCONES

INGREDIANTS:

- 1 teaspoon of cinnamon, nutmeg, allspice, cloves, or ginger, or a mixture of all
- 2 cups self-rising whole-grain flour
- 1 ounce canola margarine
- 1 cup pitted dates, chopped
- 2 tablespoons sugar
- 3/4 cup milk
- 1/2 cup skim milk powder

Method:

1) Preheat oven to 375° F.
2) Combine spices and flour, and then cut in the canola margarine. Add chopped dates, sugar, and milk. Stir until combined, then turn onto a floured cutting board and gently knead the dough.
3) Divide the dough into 2 parts and roll each into a sausage shape. Cut each dough sausage into 6 equal pieces.
4) Place pieces on a greased and floured baking sheet, spaced to allow for rising. Bake in the oven for about 8 minutes, and then reduce the temperature to 325° F and cook for another 5 to 7 minutes.

5) Serve hot. Try cutting in half and adding a light spread of canola margarine or raspberry jam on each half.

COFFEE-KISSED STEAK

Ingredients:

- 1 tablespoon ground dark-roast coffee

- ½ teaspoon kosher salt

- ½ teaspoon smoked paprika

- ½ teaspoon ground cumin

- ½ teaspoon garlic powder

- ¼ teaspoon dried thyme

- ¼ teaspoon ground cinnamon

- 2 pounds (7-bone) chuck steak

Method:

1)Combine first 7 ingredients in a bowl. Rub evenly over all sides of steak. Cover and chill 1 hour or up to 8 hours.

2) Grill over medium-high heat 3 minutes on each side or to desired degree of doneness.

CRISPY CATFISH

Ingredients:

- ¾ teaspoon salt
- 6 (4-ounce) catfish fillets
- ¼ cup hot sauce
- 2 cups crushed corn flakes
- 2 tablespoons extra-virgin olive oil

Method:

1).Sprinkle salt evenly over fish. Place in a baking dish; top with hot sauce, turning to coat all sides. Chill 1 hour.

2) Dredge fish in corn flakes. Arrange fish fillets on a baking sheet coated with cooking spray. Drizzle oil evenly over fish.

3) Bake at 425° for 10 minutes. Broil on high for 4 minutes or until golden brown and fish flakes with a fork. Serve with Collard Greens with a Kick, if desired.

GREEK-STYLE OMELET

Ingredients:

- 4 large eggs, lightly beaten
- ¼ cup chopped flat leaf parsley
- 1/8 teaspoon kosher salt
- 1/8 teaspoon freshly ground pepper
- 2 teaspoons extra-virgin olive oil
- ½ cup fresh baby spinach
- 1 plum tomato, chopped (about 1/3 cup)
- 1/3 cup crumbled feta cheese
- 8 pitted Klamath (Greek) olives, chopped

Method:

1)Whisk together first 4 ingredients.

2) Heat oil in a nonstick skillet over medium heat; add egg mixture. Cook 1 minute or until eggs begins to set.

3) Sprinkle spinach and remaining ingredients evenly over one side of egg

mixture; cover and cook 2 to 3 minutes or until spinach wilts and egg is firm. Fold side without toppings over side with toppings.

TURKEY AND SWEET PEPPER PATTIES WITH CREAMY CURRY SLAW

Ingredients:

- 1 ½ pounds boneless, skinless turkey breast, cut into 4 or 5 pieces

- 1 small onion, quartered

- 1 garlic clove

- ½ teaspoon kosher salt

- ¼ teaspoon ground red pepper

- ½ teaspoon ground cumin

- ½ red bell pepper, chopped (about 1/3 cup chopped)

- 1 tablespoon extra-virgin olive oil

Method:

1)Place turkey in the bowl of a food processor; add onion and next 4 ingredients. Grind to consistency of ground beef. Place ground chicken mixture in a bowl. Fold in chopped peppers. Shape into 4 patties. Chill 30 minutes.

2) Pour oil into a large skillet over medium-high heat. Add patties and

cook 6 or 7 minutes on each side or until thoroughly cooked. Serve with Creamy Curry Slaw.

CREAMY CURRY SLAW

INGREDIANTS:

- ½ cup Miracle Whip or mayonnaise
- 3 tablespoons apple cider vinegar
- ¼ teaspoon kosher salt
- ¼ teaspoon ground white pepper
- 1 teaspoon curry powder
- 2 tablespoons honey
- 1 (16-ounce) package coleslaw
- ½ cup chopped red onion

Method:

Whisk together Miracle Whip and next 5 ingredients in a large bowl. Add coleslaw and red onion, tossing to coat well. Chill until ready to serve.

POACHED PEAR WITH HONEY YOGURT

INGREDIANTS:

- 1 tablespoon gelatin

- 2 tablespoons hot water

- 2 cups plain yogurt

- 2 tablespoons honey

- 4 pears, peeled and halved

- Juice of 3 blood oranges

- 2 cinnamon sticks

Method:

1)Sprinkle gelatin over the hot water and let it stand for 10 minutes to soften. Mix thoroughly with the yogurt and honey.

2) Refrigerate until thickened (start preparation a few hours before needed). Place prepared pears in a saucepan.

3) Poach in blood orange juice with cinnamon sticks until fruit is soft and glowing pink, about 15 to 20 minutes.

4) Remove pears with a slotted spoon and keep warm. Boil the juice to reduce it slightly, and then remove cinnamon sticks.

5) Serve pears with the juice and the honey-thickened yogurt

OMEGA-3 BERRY SMOOTHIE

INGREDIANTS:

- 1/2 cup low-fat or skim milk—half frozen is best
- 1 tablespoon skim milk powder (can leave out if using calcium-enriched milk)
- 1 teaspoon fish* or flaxseed oil—keep bottled in refrigerator
- 1/4 cup low-fat yogurt, either plain or berry flavored (can use probiotic yogurt)
- 1/4 cup mixed berries, frozen or fresh

Method:

Using a blender, mix all ingredients together, then pour over ice if desired. Drink immediately.

Simple Vegetable, Lentil, and Tofu Soup

INGREDIANTS

- 1 clove garlic

- 1 cup pumpkin, diced

- 1 medium potato, diced

- 1 medium onion, diced finely

- 1 medium carrot, sliced finely

- 1 tablespoon canola oil

- 6 cups reduced-salt vegetable stock

- 8 ounces canned red lentils, drained

- 7 ounces firm tofu, cut into cubes

- 1 tablespoon cilantro, chopped

Method:

Sauté garlic and all the vegetables for 5 minutes in oil, stirring frequently to avoid sticking. Add the vegetable stock and lentils, and let simmer for half an hour. Add tofu just before serving. Sprinkle cilantro on top to serve.

Simple Herb Roasted Chicken

INGREDIANTS

- 1 (4-pound) whole chicken
- 2 tablespoons butter or margarine, softened
- 1 teaspoon kosher salt
- 1 teaspoon dried basil
- 1 teaspoon dried oregano
- 1 teaspoon dried rosemary
- 1 teaspoon onion powder
- 1 teaspoon smoked or Hungarian paprika

METHOD:

1) Rinse chicken inside and out and thoroughly pat dry. Using your hands, carefully detach the skin oven the chicken breast without removing skin.

2) Stir together butter or margarine and next 5 ingredients. Rub butter mixture over breast meat (under skin) covering as much surface with butter mixture as possible. Gently pull skin over chicken breast. Rub any remaining butter mixture over skin and sprinkle evenly with paprika.

3) Place chicken on a roasting rack coating with cooking spray; place rack inside a roasting pan lined with aluminum foil.

4) Bake at 350° for 45 minutes; Cover loosely with foil and bake 45 more minutes or until done. Cover, and let stand 15 minutes before carving chicken. Drizzle chicken with pan juices before serving.

CONCLUSION

Thank you for reading this full book. I have written all the information about 'Crohn's Disease'.

Don't be frustrated about Crohn's Disease. Knowledge can go a long way in treatment and

prevention.

www.ingramcontent.com/pod-product-compliance
Lightning Source LLC
Chambersburg PA
CBHW060403290526
45791CB00002B/592